Little Miss Slay

How One Makeup Artist Made Her Dreams A Reality

LING AGARAN

DEDICATION

I wrote this book for all makeup artists, hair stylists and beauty artists all over the world. To inspire, teach and show them that no dreams are too big to achieve if you really want it bad enough. To share my journey, and knowledge through business and personal experiences.

CONTENTS

ACKNOWLEDGMENTS

My Best friend Tyler - I have faced so many challenges and struggles in the past few years, but I'm pretty lucky to have an incredible person like you in my life. Thank you for the never-ending support and encouragement throughout my journey.

My coach- Michelle Stonhill- Within a year of working with you, you have given me the most valuable tools- I have developed a winning mindset, and taught me how to run a successful business.

My book strategist-Tracey Munro, I'm grateful for your friendship, and always there when I need someone to talk to. Thank you for all your hard work.

My Family:
My mom- Ethel Kump- I will always be grateful to you for bringing me to the land of opportunities.
My mom's side - The Dahilig Family- Thank you all for loving me unconditionally.

My Pro friends:
Jessica Schlamp (Jessica-Andy.ca) - Can I just say you are one talented photographer. You made me look Fab on this book cover photo.
Amine Bejjani- (Kraze Lounge)- Thank you for following me all day on my photoshoot location and making sure my hair is perfect!

Olivia Almond- my #1 cheerleader since the beginning.
(I still remember the day you stepped in to film Lashnoire when I was having a full-blown panic attack.)

Devin Almond (Nuvue Optometry) for always providing me with stylish eyewear whenever I needed.

I can't forget my best girl in the whole world:
Flora Yerxa- I'm thankful for your genuine love and friendship.

My friends, I have met along the way both personal and business, online and offline- You know who you are. Thank you for all the support.

FOREWORD

It was just over a year ago that I first encountered Ling. Within a few minutes of chatting about her vision and mission I knew that I had met someone very special.

I mentor already extraordinary women and help them to create extraordinary success in business. Ling has done what some might say is impossible. She has created an outrageously profitable business doing something that most people believe doesn't pay well, hair and makeup.

I can remember girls at school saying that they would love to train in beauty only to be told that they would never earn significant money if they did. For most beauty artists it's a tradeoff, do what you love and accept that you will never be wealthy or turn your back on a career that makes you happy and pursue something more lucrative. What if it doesn't have to be a trade off? That's the question Ling answers in this book.

Ling is living proof that you really can have it all as a beauty artist and her book is full of the lessons that will help you to get there.

I know that so many lives will be changed and new possibilities created because of this book and the woman who wrote it. I am very proud and honored to have played a small part in making it a reality.

-Michelle

LING AGARAN

CHAPTER 1
EMBRACE YOUR FLAWSOMENESS

The world is filled with people who aspire and dream. They dream about having a profession that not only pays them well, but they also want to love their work. Making your passion a reality and using it to support your life is something unique, and surely a blessing. However, some people believe that they cannot turn their dreams into a lucrative business. I beg to differ. I have always thought that everyone should try to pursue their dream profession. Hence the inspiration to write this book and tell every one of you just how important it is to believe in yourself.

It may be tough to have confidence in your ambitions as viable sources of income, but I hope to change that way of thinking by the end of this book. All of us have inspirations, dreams and goals that we wanted to achieve ever since we were children. Most of these dreams and ambitions die away with time, only to be replaced with something more realistic and more achievable. Most people have been taught that to be successful you either have to be an engineer, a doctor or a lawyer. The thing is when you believe that something is meant so fully and truly for you, you just have to go out and get it; no matter what the consequences or repercussions — taking a leap of faith, as some would call it. However, the path towards that destination is where so many people get stuck and give up. Many people will tell you that your aspirations will get you nowhere in life. But you owe it to yourself to never give up. Your ambitions should drive you to achieve it; it does not even matter if you can earn a viable income from it. At any given point in your life, you will have at least one person telling you or giving you unwanted advice, which is the complete opposite of what you want to do with your life. The trouble is that after a certain amount of time, you will start to believe that yourself.

Everyone goes through these experiences, much like me. But I was the artist of my family, the painter, the dreamer, anything but an academic. I had no interest whatsoever in becoming a doctor, nor was I ever any good at math, so there went the chances of becoming an engineer. The only thing that remained was being a lawyer, and to date, I have no idea what law is even about or how people study and learn so much. But let me tell you a bit about myself. My grandparents raised me, as my mother left to work in the Middle East when I was one. I lived in a joint family, with my aunts, uncles, and cousins, who all loved me a lot and I was very happy with them.

My mother left me in good care, with my grandparents. Since I had no father, I developed a special relationship with my grandpa. He was the father figure in my life, and I give the credit of my success to him. He was the reason I became the woman I am today.

I was born with missing fingers, and that had a limiting belief deep in my heart. How could I be successful or famous with such an abnormality? But life is ironic! I make my living now doing what I do with my hands. Anyways, so as a result of my disability, life wasn't exactly rainbows and sunshine for me.

I contracted polio at about the time my mother left me. Due to that my right leg was about twenty-two centimeters shorter than my left leg, and my foot didn't develop much either. I had to wear a brace on my right leg to help me with my walking. Add that onto my self-consciousness about being born with missing fingers and my life was just a complete shit show. Just to give you an idea of how self-conscious I was about my disabilities, I worried about what our dogs thought of me! However, I was blessed with an immensely kind and loving family, who made life pretty easy for me; they never asked me to do any of the chores my cousins had to do. I was always given special treatment, and in hindsight, that probably enabled me a lot.

I knew that someday I would have to get my leg amputated. It was a lost cause because the leg was dead. A doctor in the Philippines told me that there was no hope for my leg. I believed that man until I actually came to Canada. It was then when I realized that the people who were doctors back in the Philippines were really confident that I had about as much chance of getting my leg saved as a snowball in a forest fire. Either that or they just didn't want to be anywhere near me. However, I had to wait until I was fifteen to do that. When I was thirteen, my mom who moved to Canada from the Middle East, decided that she wanted me to live with her. Hence, she called me to Canada.

That was a very challenging time for me. I was brought up in the Philippines and didn't speak English that well when I came to Canada. Leaving my friends, family and everyone I knew behind, I moved to Canada into an entirely new culture and a new set of family as my mom had remarried. Now, I had a one-year-old half-brother. During the time I lived in the Philippines, I probably saw my mom only twice. But now we were together again. Here, my mother tirelessly looked for a doctor who could give us an alternative to amputation.

When she found a doctor, who was willing to treat me, he told me straight up that it would be very hard to treat it.

He helped me understand that amputation would be the easy way out. Or I could choose the hard way; which was to go through about five or ten extremely painful, surgical procedures. He also straight up told me that even then there was no guarantee that I would make a full recovery. Things could also go worse. I was thirteen years old then. But the decision was clear. Even if there was even a one percent chance that I would get to keep my leg, I would go for it. Turns out that was the right decision. Yes, the pain was terrible! But now my right leg is now just one-inch shorter, it's straight, and I can walk without a brace.

If I were to describe the entire process in one word, it would be 'hell.' But! I also managed to get straight A's, while on morphine (T3's) daily, dealing with that barbaric brace. I had to wear it for a few years, and it helped grow and loosen the bone. The leg had to be reconstructed using bones from my hip and left leg. That was a public battle. But there was a war raging inside of me as well. Even though I was doing well academically, I was very depressed at the time and had suicidal thoughts. It was hard enough being a teenager, in an entirely new country and I had to deal with all this pain and suffering too.

Thankfully, there was a light at the end of this dark and depressing tunnel. I got my leg back! The surgeries and the procedures went better than I could have hoped. I could hope for a brighter and more independent future now. Even though my leg was still not perfect, I learned to embrace my flaws. These experiences make me the person I am today.

Now, even though I was very grateful to have my leg back, there was still the matter of my career. As I mentioned above, the traditional professions were out of the question, and the persistent belief that being an artist will get me nowhere led me to waste ten years of my life. That is the first part of my story.

Even though I was doing administrative work, it was still somehow related to the medical field. Now it is important to consider that during the years I worked there, I was not unhappy. It was a cushy job which paid all the bills and came up with the rent as well. My basic needs were being met so there was no reason for me to be upset. However, I still was quite unhappy. I was unfulfilled, and just tired of the work and going through the same routine over and over again. The nagging thought at the back of my head told me to become an artist or at least move towards the creative field. It led me to the point where I resented having to even wake up for the day. I had known since I was fifteen that I could be a fantastic makeup artist. And it wasn't as if I wasn't already practicing those skills; I wasn't doing it as much as I would have liked. I was working on my passion part-time, and as you could expect, it was getting me nowhere taking on wedding makeup gigs on the weekends while working at the hospital for ten years.

The thing is; with a passion like this, it is either all in or nothing. I wasn't giving it my all, and there lay the reason I was unfulfilled. I had the talent, I was good at being a makeup artist, my whole life plan was made out, and even then, I was not following it. This was due to my own limiting beliefs which were a result of societal norms that led me to believe that I could never be a rich-ass makeup artist. Society thinks that those who have made it in this industry are there due to a stroke of luck. However, if you see some of the most famous people in this industry, they are at that level because they never gave up on their dream.

They just did what made them happy and what satisfied them. In my case, I knew what would make me happy, and satisfy me. However, responsibilities came in the way of me pursuing my dreams. I had to pay my rent; I had to pay for utilities, groceries, and everything else in between.

My cushy nine to five job enabled me to do all of that. It provided me with the security of knowing exactly where my next paycheck was going to come from, and the thought of leaving that made me scared. I am actually very grateful for that job because in a way that made me financially stable enough to get a business going in the first place and of course pay my way through. However, the fact that I had limiting beliefs that stopped me from pursuing what I knew, in my hearts of heart, would fulfill me.

Happiness is not easy to attain. It is one thing to imagine yourself already having achieved your goal, and it is another thing altogether to work towards that goal and make it into a reality. This is exactly where all those metaphors about hard work come from. I won't pretend as if getting to that point was all sunshine and rainbows, however being where I am today was worth all the entire painful journey. I have noticed that most people are scared of hard work. It's just that they don't know if that hard work, all the pain, sweat, and tears, will even pay off. They are not able to face failure or do not like to venture on the unknown. They are scared to take the risk of "*what if*".

Attaining happiness isn't just about doing what makes you happy. It is so important to enjoy your passion first, so you actually get a taste for it. You realize that if you're good enough to actually gain proficiency in your passion, then you'd definitely be able to find a way to make money doing it. The fact is that if you're good enough at what you do, money will automatically follow. The fact of the matter is that if you're following your passion without making money it's really just a money pit.

The struggle is very real in the practical world, which is why most people don't ever take that leap of faith. They don't know the pay off at the end. Especially in my field, most makeup artists work full-time jobs along with carrying on their passion. It is entirely understandable that they do so. However, it is not ideal. They, much like me, have let society tell them that they cannot turn their passion into a lucrative business.

Every day going into my administrative job felt like I was doing something I wasn't meant to do. It just felt wrong having something that I was so good at and passionate about and working as an administrator. Each passing year I thought about quitting and working full time as a makeup artist. However, that didn't stop me from doing everything I could to give a 110% at my job at the hospital. I actually cared about helping people and playing a role in people's lives. I did get some satisfaction from it, but then again it wasn't my passion nor my purpose. But I had convinced myself already that this is something that just couldn't be done. And this is where most people get stuck. Just thinking about what you want to achieve gives you some pleasure and most people are okay with that slight vision of success.

My job and passion gave me a sense of accomplishment. Yet I knew when I was working at the hospital that this wouldn't be enough for me. I was battling between wanting to pursue my passion and being scared of leaving. I was just scared of failing so much so that I put a hold on it for the longest time. I didn't want to end up in a position where I couldn't even support myself. It was frustrating, I knew that I would leave someday, but that day just wasn't coming. When the time did come to leave this job, I was doing it because I realized that if I stayed I would not be living up to my full potential and creating the life that I desired. I knew that if I stayed on any longer, I would turn into a really miserable cow. And that was exactly what happened. I started to get really snappy and sensitive in the end. That was when I knew I needed to get the fuck out.

Envisioning yourself already having achieved what you want brings some short-lived satisfaction. However, turning that idea into reality takes strength and conviction. It is not easy for anyone, as it wasn't for me. Every day for ten years straight I had to go into a job that just wasn't my passion.

The only thing I looked forward to was the coming weekend when I knew that I would be working on my part-time job, being a makeup artist. Those two days spent working as a make-up artist brought me more satisfaction than the other five days doing administrative work at my job.

My passion became plan B instead of plan A. It was more of a hobby than anything else, and it was an expensive hobby at that. On top of that, it wasn't even a hobby I could make money from.

That was the trouble with what I was going. If I could not make my hobby into something I could make money from then, it was just money down the drain. My cushy job, which was enough to support me was certainly not enough to support me and my hobby in the long term. Finally, when I hit the eight-year mark at my job, I had had enough. I had started thinking of quitting my job at that time. In hindsight, I knew that it was high time that I took a step towards it. However, I still didn't do it due to fear and not believing in myself. I just felt like this wasn't the purpose of my life, I felt it in my bones, and I knew that I would not be doing myself any justice if I continued down this road. At this point in my life, I was willing to do just about anything to make my hobby more lucrative.

So, I decided one day that I would leave my job and pursue my passion full time. I had had enough of stress and unhappiness, the only two things I felt at my current job when I realized that I shouldn't be there any longer. I realized that I should go out and chase my dreams. I was never the sort of person who would settle for anything less than what they wanted, but it took me ten years to realize that that is precisely what I had been doing. However, when I did grasp it, it was with the full conviction that it was indeed time to make something of myself, doing things I loved.

Finally, I decided to ask for a six-month sabbatical, so that I could focus more on my passion. However, my request was denied, but I wasn't giving up. A few weeks later, I put in another request for a sabbatical, and this time it was for one year, and by some miracle, it was approved! I didn't know what they were thinking, denying one request and approving the other one, but I am thankful for my stars that they did!

Of course, as it turned out, they were very supportive of me and gave me one year to make it work. They knew that this wasn't my passion, to be working at the hospital for the rest of my life; I still felt a bit sad to be leaving all my friends and the doctors and nurses I've worked with for ten years. But at the same time very excited, happy and peaceful to be pursuing my dream, even though I was scared shitless. In my last year at the office, I applied for a leave that would help me go over my thoughts. Staying back for those two years made me quite unhappy, however, on some level, it must have provided me with the security I needed too. I felt like my passion was slipping away, bit by bit every day. Two years of fear held me back thinking I could not make it out there and I had no confidence in myself. How the fuck would I pay my bills?

That coupled with the nagging doubt of if I am good enough to make it in the world?

Now it is essential to understand the gravity of the decision I had just made. I had just decided to leave a cushy job that paid all of my bills and supported me in a vocation that did nothing for my financial status. In that situation, when you have already made the decision and committed yourself to act upon it, you do have to tell yourself to calm down. Otherwise, you would be in a complete panic, thinking about how you are going to support yourself. I told myself that I was still young and even if turning my passion into a lucrative business didn't work out, I could still make money, somehow.

That being said, I had a secure job at the hospital for a year, and I could always go back to it. Since my plan B had now become my plan A, I needed another plan B. It was also nice having someone with me who was there to support me through the tough times and help me turn my dream into a reality. He gave me emotional support and was there for me when I needed. However, deep in my heart I knew the path I must follow to attain happiness and satisfaction but I feared what was to come. But that didn't mean that I wouldn't follow that path, no matter what the circumstances. I was scared deep down, but even deeper down I knew I had the confidence to make this decision and land on my feet, no matter what. I just needed a little bit of a push from him, his support was very important to me. Despite it all, it had been a tough decision, especially considering that I had gone ten years without wondering how I was going to support myself.

So, to summarize it, I knew I wanted to build a lucrative business. But more importantly, I wanted to live and love life, wake up every day with excitement and fire, creating the life that I loved. I understood that money is just a byproduct of my passion. I know that when I have the intention of serving my clients and enjoying my job, the money will follow. I know if I live my passion, then I can manifest anything I want and have all the abundance in life. However, it was the question of wanting it enough and convincing myself that everything I had heard throughout my life could be proven wrong through hard work.

This took me ten years to realize and was the second step. The third was putting that idea into action and taking practical steps into making it a reality, which was leaving my job and actually working towards my goal. The day I took a leave of absence from my job, I knew that I did not have another second to waste. After leaving I realized that even though I wanted to be a makeup artist, I still had no plan whatsoever. I had only thought as far as leaving my job. Just that decision took so much courage and so much space in my mind that I forgot to think about actually planning out what I was going to do next, and more importantly, how I will get paid. Leaving my job was purely a leap of faith, and when I realized this, I said the one thing that everyone says to themselves in that sort of situation. *'Whatever happens, happens.'*

However, it wasn't all talk and no show. Now that I had left my job, I had to get down to business and do something about my business. The funny thing is, when you have spent, nearly a decade thinking about something and building it up in your head, you do have some idea what you are doing. So, at this point, I just decided that I was going to take charge of it all. I was already a skilled makeup artist; however, I had no business. For my passion to be a viable business I needed to have clients and I needed to have a brand. This was the time for action. I did know that the first way to capture business was to make a name of myself, because if nobody knows you, why are they going to come to you? So, I had to market myself, and the first thought that popped into my mind was social media. I made pages all over every social media platform I could think of and also started to make connections with everyone I could get a hold of in the industry. I still had a lot to learn about operating my own business, and I knew that I could not go long without having some income to support myself.

I gave myself a year to make it. Now, I know that that sounds very unrealistic and childish, however, the sort of situation I was in, I could not allow myself any more time. I did everything I could during that time. I made connections with people who were more business savvy than me, and I started to learn from them. I found out that for any business to be a viable and lucrative source of income, I had to manage the creative part as well as the annoying part. I had to manage the books, crunch the numbers, have a growth plan, and create a website for potential clients to visit: these were just a few things on my ever-growing list of things that needed to get done to make my business successful. I had so much left to learn and implement that I knew that resting was not an option. If I was in this business, I had to be all in. Otherwise,

I would not be in it at all. Finding out just how little I knew about actually running a business is where reality set in.

As I mentioned above, nobody in my family is an entrepreneur except my grandpa. He was a businessman, but he passed away before I could get an understanding of what he did. As such, I had no idea what it took to start a business or keep it afloat. This realization left me thinking that I couldn't do it at all and that was a heart-crushing realization. However, since I was not going to give up without giving it my all, I buckled down and studied.

LING AGARAN

CHAPTER 2

DARE TO DREAM

I had lived a life of painful exclusion. I was always the outsider, the other person. My days at school had been depressing. I couldn't play with my classmates, and they couldn't relate to my dilemma. However, it would all be over soon. My surgeries had been successful, and I was grateful to be alive and well. The surgical procedures had caused quite a lot of pain and torment. I was glad to have made it through. My legs were almost the same length now. The pain of surgeries was well worth it. I got much more than I was hoping for.

Life resumed as usual after the surgeries were over. I got back to my ambitions and completed my studies. I knew that a good education would enable me to have a good life, a good job and make money. That is really all anyone asks for, and I made those goals a reality. I wasn't about to give up on them.

I had a really interesting educational background. I attended a private college and majored in tourism management. That was only because I didn't really know what I wanted yet. It was almost like a buffer until I figure out what I really want.

After finishing college, I quickly realized that was not where I needed, or wanted, to be. Due to this uncertainty, I gave it a rest for a while and switched jobs, one to the next. They were all so boring and uninspiring. I got fired a lot or I quit; and when I say I quit, I meant like staying in a job for no more than two weeks at a time. I had the attention span of a two-year-old and kept going from one job to the next. I obviously couldn't really keep a job. This made me wonder if something was wrong with me.

Finally, I was tired of moving from job to job. Everyone around me started to criticize me and question why I always was getting fired or quitting. I had no answer except that it wasn't challenging, it wasn't inspiring, nor did it light up my life. I was the person who woke up every day, just dreadful because I had to go to work. However, I eventually had to just force myself to grow up, pick a career and stick with it.

Since I was convinced that I could never make money from my passion, I put it at the back of my head. I finally settled in the medical health field. Yes, yes...I know it is so obvious. But I wasn't getting any younger so I picked a career that is safe, and would support my life. It wasn't necessarily the lifestyle I wanted, but good enough to live a normal life; pay my living expenses and maybe go on a trip a year. So, went to college again, choosing Nursing Unit Assistant and got a good job at the hospital getting settled into my 9-5 job. I was always told that's how it works. We get the diplomas and degrees, use them to get a cushy job with chances of future growth, and ultimately settle down into that life. At least that's how it worked in my family. I did my best to do the same. I had the education and the job, but I did not have the fulfillment these achievements were supposed to bring. I was not meant for this life. I was good at it, and that is an understatement. I really excelled at it. My work ethic stayed the same even after I had made up my mind to leave the hospital to pursue my dreams. To be honest, this is actually my pet peeve, people getting the job and not caring for the work they're doing. My mentality was clear; do the job you're given and do it right otherwise don't do it at all. Just because you don't love the job you have doesn't mean you have to half-ass through the day. I always did my job, going above and beyond what was expected of me; for the people I worked for and the people I worked with. My life worked like freaking clockwork; work, home, eat, look forward to weekend and repeat. Don't get me wrong here, there is nothing wrong with this. In fact, people who are able to do this are exceptionally well maintained and have a much more settled life. Unfortunately, I did not want this predictive style for myself. My gut kept telling me that I was meant to do more than this.

No matter how much I tried, the feelings of desolation and absolute dread would come back in full force. I didn't want to be called difficult or ungrateful because the job was paying me more than the industry average. However, I was meant for a different life.

I desperately tried to hold on to the idea I was leading a normal life, and that the unhappiness was just a part of growing up. This was the life that society expected me to lead. I believed what society wanted me to believe; I was just as normal as I could be. I had achieved the first part of the societal norm. I got a job! Hoo-fucking-ray. Doing everything that society wanted me to do meant putting away my passion for being a makeup artist. I ignored how I felt about my life. I thought I was being greedy about wanting more than what I had.

That caused a lot of personal pain. Living through that for many years taught me one fundamental lesson. If you want to be better, it's not greed. If you are satisfying your need for a more rewarding life and doing what you want to do, then you are just fulfilling your destiny. I didn't know it.

I'd like to address people who say you should be happy with what you have… to them I ask; how can you ever be happy if your life is the exact thing that is making you unhappy? If you don't do things that make you happy, you will inevitably feel stuck, and that won't change unless you pursue what makes you feel alive and grateful. The saying, 'the heart wants what it wants,' applies well to this situation.

Although I had a seemingly normal life, in reality, I was living a nightmare. I had convinced myself that my career as a Nursing Unit Assistant was all I needed. I made myself believe like it was my calling to work in the medical field since I spent most of my young adult life in the hospital. I tried to distract myself from the pain I felt within, by practicing empathy with the patients. That is how my passion, my true calling became my Plan B. I had convinced myself that I couldn't turn my love into a money-making career. Had you told me then, that I would become an entrepreneur and do those very things, I would have laughed in your face!

However, after working at the hospital for eight years, I had this nagging feeling I wanted to do more in life. The norms of society I held so dear became less important. Life had become dreary and the being okay with working on my passion on the weekends was not enough anymore. I knew in my hearts of hearts that this was not what I wanted to do with my life. However, I couldn't exactly just up and leave. I had to look after myself and provide for myself. So, dreary or not, I still had to do it. Sometimes you are just so set in your ways. The comfort that those ways provide, that to change seems next to impossible.

You fear what might happen if you are not good enough, or capable enough or what if you go all in on this one thing, and lose it all? You see failure all around you, everything and everyone seems to stop you from doing what you want to do. You recall memories of the times you tried to do something, and you failed and the only question you can ask yourself, every time you so much as think about quitting and taking the plunge, is 'what if I don't make it?'

That fear; that self-doubt, is so gripping that you can spend an entire life trying to overcome it. Even if you make it and get to the top of your field, that fear and self-doubt never really go away. They are always there, nagging at you; however, you learn how to control it. You learn to channel that fear into something positive. I have learned time and time again that you are only as good as you allow yourself to be. If you think you aren't worth shit, well then, guess what? You aren't worth shit. All the people I have met over the years; successful people from my industry and others, they all had the same beginning. They could envision themselves succeeding. They knew that they were worth it and that they deserved it. You can take the example of the greatest bodybuilder of all time, Arnold Schwarzenegger:

"If I had listened to the naysayers, I would still be in the Austrian Alps, yodeling."

And all of that is well and true. However, I might have a biased opinion. The thing is after you reap the fruit of the struggles; you forget just how difficult the journey was. You have already put in the hard work; you have made the climb, and now you are relaxing and living your best life. That time in my life was a blessing in disguise. Though I did not know it then.

Throughout the years I worked in the hospital, I could not stop thinking about it. My passion festered so profoundly within me that I never stopped thinking about it. I wanted it so bad I would often daydream about going back home so I could learn to improve myself or just have fun; ya know? *'When you are doing something you love, it doesn't seem like work.'* Let me tell you, I was 'never working on the weekends. However, again it was just plain anguish, wanting something else when you already have an alternative which is plain and easy.

I was making decent money at the hospital and wanting to do something else was just torture.

Why would I want more when I have it good and easy? Why am I playing small? Why am I scared so badly? This work that I was doing was certainly not something that I was passionate about. I was doing it so I could pay for my bills.

These questions ran rampant in my mind every day and every time I came up with an answer for any of them, I had only one thought.

What. Is. The. Worst. That. Can. Happen!

Honestly think about it, if you were to chase your dream, *what is the worst-case scenario? You lose your job!* Well, there will always be a next one. *You'll have to move into a smaller apartment to save on expenses!* You'll buy an even bigger house when you are successful. *You'll have to work hard?* Well, what else did you think life was about?

This is the present me talking. The old me was scared shitless of these questions. Sure, I can console myself now that I have a successful business. However, back then no matter how much I loved and cherished my dream, my fear always overtook me. It won over and over again. *What do I know about business? Who the hell am I to think I can be a successful makeup artist and a female entrepreneur badass warrior?*

Well, the last one was a stretch, but you know where I'm going with this, right?

I was losing by miles, to my fears. My passion took a back seat and only became a dream. I had turned my passion into a hobby instead of a career I love. My scarcity mindset won.

LING AGARAN

CHAPTER 3

REACH FOR THE LASH

My family taught me a lot about money quite early on in life. Since I lived with my grandparents, they were filled with advice on how to live a life with a steady financial flow. Looking at them I knew that I had to have a stable life that was as good as them. I decided that I would save a percentage of my hard-earned money. I vowed to myself that I would never spend that money until I needed to invest in something or was old and retired. Even though following this process is just about the most boring thing ever! But it made sense because when rainy days come, they pound hard on you!

I did just that and saved a percent of my income. Now you would think this plan would have gone towards me making it in my makeup artist business, and you would be right, that is if I hadn't already spent it all on a business venture before deciding to leave my job. This happened about a year before I left my job. When I finally was free from the mundane work routine, I tried to figure out what I was supposed to do. I knew I had to do something that would inspire me to strive harder every day and I knew that something related to the beauty industry would bring forth that inspiration in me. But I had no idea what specification I was going to pursue. It could be anything from a make-up related product that I could invest in or a skin care product, or even start my beauty salon. Through trial and error, I realized that there was one thing that irked me the most, which the current fake eyelashes were being sold in the market. To me, they looked very artificial and plastic. I thought to myself that there was a need to have better lashes in the market. If I could make better eyelashes and sell them, then this was going to be a good business idea.

While I was working solo on this idea, I didn't think of the prospects it held for me, all I knew was that I am going to make a better product. From there on, I included a few people in my team to make the eyelashes, and in a matter of a few months, we were thinking about creating an entire line of lashes. My amazing idea was to call it Lashnoire – a premium stripped lash product, and I had created it. I know, I know. Impressive, right? But unfortunately for me, I did something, and it didn't turn out the way I wanted it to.

When this happened, I was taken aback. Time and money were spent, and it didn't give a fruitful result.

But let me tell you, that entire process was perhaps one of the best experiences of my life. The story of Lashnoire is one of an incredible journey, a painful one at that. Anyway, years ago, I would do my bridal makeup 'gig' over the weekend lashes was becoming a thing, and I knew it was here to stay. The thing was, the quality of the eyelashes that were coming in was something I hated. The quality of the stripped lashed back then was terrible. They were cheap, plastic-y, and weighed heavily on the eyelid.

I hated using it on bridal makeup jobs, it would cheapen my work, and the worst part was that it didn't even look good. In bridal makeup, everything was so detailed that the lashes just destroyed the image. Since I love focusing on the eyes on any person I am doing make up for, lashes were a big concern for me. Since they were so heavy, the stripped lashes often fell out. There was no way in hell I was letting my clients walk around like that when they say their 'I do's.' Now, I might sound like I have little of unresolved anger issues there and I might. Those preposterous things were abominable! Anyway, I digress. Long story short, with Lashnoire I researched for quality lashes, and to my great displeasure, I found nothing that made me even remotely happy. Nothing that would make me go wow, nor anything that made me excited. I don't exactly remember how I got into it, but I suppose it was something along the line of hatred fueled rage against the stripped lashes. I knew I needed to make my job, easier by having simple eyelashes that do not take a lot of time to apply. Before these lashes, I often found myself compromising on the eye makeup I did on my clients.

If there is one thing that absolutely stands out in my personality, it is the fact that I am an ambitious and determined person. Rather than how I am facing a setback, I focus more on solving the problem. In fact, I won't stop until I find a solution for it. When it came to the eyelashes, I was yet again obsessed with finding a more natural way to wear eyelashes. I always think that you can have anything and everything you want and a firm believer of that theory that the world is my oyster. Anyway, the next thing I know, I'm researching manufacturers capable of mimicking the real shape and (hair) of eyelashes. During my research, I found ten manufacturers. From those ten manufacturers, I started by eliminating the least favorite ones and eventually ended up with just three. I then took upon creating and designing the products. However, I should clarify that I had no intention of putting it out there at first. I did not expect that this could become a business, but I was determined to do what I wanted. I think around this time I was more excited about the fact that I have stashed of personal goodies for my clients and me. I had no clue how to market this or how people even get it out. That wasn't my concern then. I was just excited that I could create. I knew then that this validated my love for makeup and anything to do with beauty. If I was unsuccessful in my previous attempt and if I had to go over the entire process again, I would. I just enjoyed the process. I was very interested in the artistic side of creating. It started as a hobby, and once I had decided on what type of hair I wanted to use, I went into designing my lashes, which eventually came to be known as Lashnoire.

On a side note, it would amaze you to find out how many of your hobbies you can turn into something that can help you earn a good amount of money. Lashnoire didn't start that way, but I knew I could make it profitable. All I needed was proper guidance and an actual business model to do it. You have to know which opportunity to grab and when. Anyway, I kept makeup artists, clients and myself in mind as I designed. For our clients, I wanted something that was durable, and mimicked actual eyelashes that looked fluffy, instead of looking like something taken off of Barbie. I wanted them to be weightless and look amazing in photographs as well. Obviously, to achieve all these things, I had to make sure they were luxury and a premium quality.

Now, with big jobs, like bridal makeup, the makeup artists usually had to manage time to get the job done. They had other things on their plate as well and needed material that could be used effectively and efficiently. For professional makeup artists, every second and every minute counts, I wanted the lashes to fit the curve of the client's eye shape. Like DUH! Lashnoire would be a success! I was golden; I had lashes that would make everyone's eyes look fab!

That helped me in making multiple designs to fit every eye shape. Lashnoire has styles for all eye shapes. This idea was what gave birth to the tagline *"fatally flawless"*. When I made multiple designs for different eye shapes, I started out with my own eyes. When I was designing these eyelashes, I had to keep in options for natural to dramatic looks. I eventually ended up creating six styles, and that was probably the most fun I had. I went back and forth with the manufacturer, and it actually felt like I was running a business; making a product that would help countless other makeup artists and me with their work, while ensuring that my clients looked beautiful. I became super detailed with the eyelashes I was designing, everything had to be perfect.

The length, weight, volume in each lash had to be just right. Then they had to be tested so they wouldn't harm the skin. My main USP (unique selling proposition) was simple; make my client's eyes look stunning. These lashes could also be used 20 times, which is not offered by most eyelash brands. I made sure that I covered every nook and cranny. This was my baby, metaphorically! I had to make sure that it was perfect. You name it, I had thought of it, all of it. All of this became my life and baby for about a year.

From dreaming about it to researching, designing and launching it, everything was a point of concern for me. When I finally reached the end stage, and I had the final product in front of my eyes, I was ecstatic. I had designed these fantastic lashes, and immediately after the ecstasy, I felt blue. What do I do now? One year of my life and now I was done with it. Was I supposed to put these in my closet and never think of them again and only bring them out to admire them? I talked this through with Tyler. He was the one person that went with all my crazy ideas no matter how far-fetched they were. There had been multiple times that after listening to my crazy ideas, sometimes he would look at me with blank eyes, like what sort of crazy is it going to come out of Ling's make-believe land this time? But despite my ideas, he would still help me, and understandably he was with me through my entire crazy phase. We went back and forth with it until I realized what I wanted to do with it.

I came to this realization and wanted to go for it full-time and share it with the world and hence the birth of Lashnoire. I was going through with it and that my product would be out for the rest of the world to use. I think this was the second step of my career, the first being leaving my job of almost a decade. When I started Lashnoire, I still hadn't left my job, and I wasn't precisely struggling on the money front. I had a full-time job along with good savings, thanks to the boring yet reliant method of saving for rainy days. I used those savings to start of Lashnoire.

The worst part about starting a business is that so much goes into it that there is no way that a novice like me could have made a successful model out of this. The marketing agency helped me in no way achieve my dreams. They didn't deliver on their promise, and actually tried to make me do what they were supposed to be doing in the first place. If you have ever started a business, you probably know how a marketing agency operates. Their first instinct is to secure the client, and in my case, they did this by promising me the world and showing me the stars. They promised to help me get Lashnoire off the ground and make it into a viable business model.

Even though I could see no results, and simultaneously see my money going down the drain, I could not fire them. I was already too far into it, and I believed that I needed them.

The feeble hope I had, making this into a viable business was so firmly attached to me, that I justified their failures by convincing myself that this was my career. I had enough money, and I could always make more money. That was a small price to pay for my career. Besides, I figured there's no turning around with Lashnoire now, we are about to launch this product, and I knew something wasn't right with it. I could see the marketing agency had no solid plan.

I took about three months to understand that things were not progressing as they were supposed to. The communication was off; they didn't believe in me as an artist; we had the meetings after meetings, discussing the same shit over and over again. They were like monkeys in suits, well dressed, smiling but no clue about what was going on. I was furious, frustrated and anxious at the same time. That is a dangerous combo. I was in a blinding rage all the time, and I couldn't say anything to the people making me angry because I needed them. The thought of paying for this shit show made me even more hopeless.

It all came back to me. I remembered all the things that the naysayers had said to me about being a makeup artist just being an expensive hobby, one that would never make me any considerable money. Now scarcity sets in again. But unlike the last time where I had little to lose, there was actually a business and a lot of money on the line, and I was scared it was going to fail before it even started. My gut feeling was the strongest it had ever been, I remember always being up all night, crying, working but not accomplishing anything. Just worried sick.

The people at the marketing agency I had hired told me they couldn't market me and I had to do that myself once the product was ready to be launched. I could not figure out for fuck's sake why I was paying them shit tons of money. Anytime I would ask them regarding the progress of my work they would either be unavailable or if they would even answer my calls, they would be unsupportive of my ideas. I was so stressed that I think I had a nervous breakdown. I don't remember a time before this, where I had such a hard time dealing with people. I started to believe that Lashnoire was the problem.

They couldn't do much, but they did give me a vital life lesson. They gave me the motivation to learn. Indirectly, because of them I was forced to learn how to do it myself. I learned marketing on my own. I realize all of this when I look back at that time. I let them go four months later. In hindsight, that was probably one of the best learning experiences I ever had. *"Failure is just the opportunity to begin again, this time more intelligently." -Henry Ford*

In the annals of failures, starting again is hard to do... even visualizing yourself in a position where you can start over is hard to do. Back then, I felt so angry and lost on Lashnoire. It had sunk even before it had the chance to start. I didn't even want to take the name 'Lashnoire' again. I had used every bit of my savings on taking this brand off the ground. It left me penniless and on the verge of depression. Damn near it.

I blamed myself, there goes Ling, making a fool of herself again. Another epic failure in her life. You know those inspirational stories of people who believed in their business against all the odds and got it off the ground? Stories of companies like FedEx, Netflix or many world-class brands..yeah, I wasn't them. But if they could do it, so could I.

Eight months later, I decided to stop feeling shitty about what happened. To be honest I thought that was part of the struggle. I was right on at least one front. I got back up and marketed on my own. I learned about the ins and outs, researched my competitions, networked with other people in the industry, and pushed my product on the back of

YouTube, Instagram influencers, sponsored designers, and also had my own YouTube channel.

I got my hands on just about anything I could use to get the product out there. I got my mojo back when I saw that makeup artists and beauty influencers loved the quality of Lashnoire. For the first time in so fucking long, I fell back in love with Lashnoire. That painful experience with the marketing agency all of that happened for a reason. I know now that whatever happened, happened for a reason. I had to go through that and live with that to make me tougher and prepare me to become what I am now. I have to go through everything because all of that taught me something; everything had a purpose.

Now, Lashnoire is a great product I can offer to my clients, beauty artists and beauty influencers alike. The trouble was that it was getting harder to quit the full-time job that supported my bills and my life. It was tough to jump ship and quit the job at the hospital. Lashnoire gave me hope that maybe, just maybe I was on the right path. Lashnoire gave me a glimpse of what it would be like to be a boss bitch! And boy, let me tell you, I loved that. I freaking loved that feeling, and I could not let go of that feeling. Even then I couldn't deny how I itched to go out and attain that feeling again. People close to me saw that change in my personality. In both happiness and misery, whichever way you want to look at it. However, just when I was on the top of the world and working hard to market my lash brand, things weren't going well at work. I had an emotional breakdown which caused me to ask for a stress leave to take care of myself. They granted me a two-week stress leave. The thing was that maybe it all getting to be a bit too much for me. However, instead of hating the situation, I decided instead to focus on the pros and cons of staying at my job or quitting it. I like to refer to this point as the 'make it or break it' because logic and desire go so strongly against each other that you have to decide. You either say fuck it and go all in, or you give it up. Logically, quitting my job for a career in makeup artistry was a bad idea. I was in a financially stable position and leaving that for a chance of making it was not at all right. I had a safe job. When this happens your mind and heart are in a constant battle every minute, of every day. You look at the person you are closest to, who has seen you cry, laugh, in doubt, in insecurity, and you question your whole worth and purpose. Bringing problems home from work and staying at a job I no longer loved or enjoyed. Now that also affects your personal life.

The thing is, everyone has their limits. The problems I was going through had now changed my relationships as well.

When that happens, it hits you. Sort of like an epiphany. I had to make a choice. Here I would like to stress that every one of us has an opportunity. I did as well. I had two clear cut options in front of me, I could either take the risk, or I could play it safe for the rest of my life. It was a leap of faith, with no plan but I had to take a stab at being an entrepreneur.

I didn't even know what it meant to be an entrepreneur and whenever I pictured myself in that position; it was like seeing a chicken running around with its head cut off. But there's this thing we call 'heart.' That bastard is hard to ignore. It was so unbearable that I could feel physical anguish over my decision. I reflected on what had happened with Lashnoire, and all those signs were clear. They were telling me to be ballsy and ask for a leave of absence. My two weeks of stress leave had given me a chance to clear my head and do what was best. The universe had my back once again.

I knew without a doubt, after the two weeks stress leave, that I needed to get back to work and the first thing I needed to do was ask for a leave of absence. I had waited long enough, and I now needed to feed my soul. I knew that wouldn't be happening at my job at the hospital. I needed to stop dreaming and take action on that dream.

I didn't have a shit's worth of an idea what that entailed, but I knew that I would figure it out. I would cross that bridge when I got to it. That decision is very hard. It's bittersweet because you are either standing on a potential goldmine or you are doomed. I knew in my heart that my life was about to change and I was ready for the good, the bad and the ugly. I made the most critical decision. It was unknown what was to come of that decision, but I then had the courage and the one person believing in me to make it all happen. That was all the validation I needed at that point.

"The rest would fall into place, and it was not worth worrying about anyway." Ling Agaran

CHAPTER 4
MAKE MAGIC HAPPEN

Dreams are always outrageous and farfetched. If they aren't, then you aren't dreaming big enough. Your thoughts, ambitions, and aspirations should scare you. They should be bigger than your life. It is very similar to that metaphor, *"Aim for the moon, even if you miss you'll land on the stars."* If you ask me, the stars are pretty cool too. The hardest part of making your dreams become a reality is to go after them with all you have. Especially when you decide to be a makeup artist because then you are being told by everyone repeatedly that your dreams are crazy, stupid and it would be silly to pursue them.

One of my many limiting beliefs was, being a wedding makeup artist, was not enough to pay the bills or make it full time. Weddings are seasonal and there was no way I could live with such little chances of income. That was silly talk. There is no such thing as a seasonal wedding. I just didn't know where to find more clients and I had no solid marketing plan then.

The opinions of others started to make sense. These opinions instill a fear of the unknown within us. Hearing such motivating things makes deciding and getting your shit together harder than it should be. A handful of people cannot let what others say affect them. They are amazing, to be honest, because it is one of the hardest things to do. Words can hurt, and it's difficult to ignore them when they are coming from people you value the most.

Even harder than that is when you are standing at the brink of deciding, and you don't know what lies on the other end. Because you have spent your entire life practically without even knowing what you will do when you are following your passion. You can see the right side, which is your success, but you can never envision the entire journey. No matter how hard you try, no matter how much you have thought it over, when you are standing at the edge of the tunnel, you always feel you are unprepared. That is because you are. However, you need to feel the need to do this one thing in life, brim up to your throat and explode. That one thing is:

"Grab life by the balls."

It is literally that simple, and still complex at the same time. Because life is pretty good at guarding its balls, you see.

The hardest part for me was going through the tunnels of the unknown, not even knowing if I would ever reach the other side, ever. But I decided I will follow the pearls of wisdom mentioned above. When I finally opened to people about my dreams and aspirations, they gave me this look that made me think if I was asking for unicorns, rainbows, and a selfie with Bigfoot and then came the comments that demotivated me.

However, the one thing that stood by me was my ego. Most people think that ego is a bad thing. However, I would like to disagree. I am not talking about the 'fuck all of you, I am better than all of you,' attitude. Instead, I am talking about the ego that lights a fire under your ass, makes you look at the tunnel and go, 'Ya know what. That doesn't seem impossible.' It's kind of like that Japanese proverb, *"If one can do it, then I can do it. If no one can do it, then I must do it."* That ego feeds the need to prove myself would help me leave no stone unturned in my quest to prove myself. I want what I want regardless of how many times and how many people tell me I cannot do it. My ego is everything to me since I started this business.

It had led me up to the point of getting me to stand at the edge of the tunnel, light a massive fire up my ass and then made me run. I knew I was ready; it was fucking go time!

Let me tell you, when I entered that tunnel, I was ready to do everything it took to get to the end. I was not scared of putting in hours spent working hard. I didn't really have many distractions or things that needed my time, and even if I did, this took precedence.

I was willing and excited to put aside sleep, and spend that time learning new skills, which would lead me to the end of the tunnel. When I quit my job, I made sure I was ready to put in my all. Every fiber of my being had to be dedicated to making my business a success and keep going until I could not go on anymore. Let me tell you, that point is a long way off and for me, it seemed as if it would never come. I was ready to sacrifice each and everything and be committed to my business. Even though that might sound as if all of this happened overnight, it is quite the opposite.

I was not going to burn myself out right at the beginning. I had to pace myself and take it one step at a time. I asked myself what I needed to do every day to move closer to my dreams. The answer came in the form of this quote I once read, and it has stuck with me ever since.

"Figure out who you want to be, what you want to do, what inspires you and gets you up in the morning, and then figure out how you can get there and what it takes to be that person."

Having dreams and aspiration is not enough. It is the bare minimum to get started, to be honest. In all honesty, all jokes aside, this quote became my starting point when I left my job. I had done just about every type of thinking there needed to be done so I could make it to what I wanted to be. I wanted to be the person with who could describe herself in the following words.

"Hello, my name is Ling Agaran. I am a sought-after makeup artist who specializes in luxury weddings."

Boy, I couldn't wait to say this to people and know in my hearts of heart it is true. I could not wait for that time to come. This was for the world. For me, I wanted my motivation to get me up in the morning to be my passion. I wanted to go to sleep knowing that I will have a full schedule and many clients the next day. I tried to do what I loved, meet new people, and make them look pretty, confident and the best version of themselves. That really revved up my engines.

Imagining all of that was well and good, but then reality came into play. How in the bloody hell am I going to start, never mind even get to that point? Yeah...this realization hit me like a ton of bricks. As soon as I had quit my job, all my dreams of giving it my all and grabbing life by the balls went right out the window for a second. I wondered if I should beg for my job back, wondering if I was in over my head. The reality of the situation hits and I think I have just left my job with no idea how to get from point A to point B. I had to stop second-guessing myself, and I needed to get on track. To do that, I had to remind myself that,

"Everything you want is on the other side of fear."

I cannot put into words the jubilation I felt when that was all it took to stop these thoughts from driving me nuts. When these negative thoughts take hold over you, you look the part too. This did not go unnoticed by the surrounding people. They wondered if I was going crazy having a conversation with myself. When you make random gestures and get vacant looks over your face, people ask questions, the answers to which you seek too. I questioned my self-esteem. The nagging voice in your head that keeps you down became strong, whispering in my ears, 'you're just a local makeup artist in a small town in Canada BC.'

Eventually, these doubts and questions piled up, and I was frustrated for not knowing how to solve the problems I was facing. Nor was I any close to getting any answers. I had a full-on panic induced talk with myself where I asked myself these questions and with no answers to console myself with; I became worse and worse. Each time was harder than the one before. I had the mislead misconception I would get somewhere in life once I quit my job. Fair warning to those who are about to go through this, or are already going through this, when your fears and self-doubts kick in again, in those moments you need to hold firmly to the belief that you will make it. You need to work on your mindset. Part of me knew that I would make it big enough. However, there was also another part that was filled with fears and doubts. However, the power that your dreams hold eventually prevail over your doubts. I did ultimately achieve that, and I have been comfortable for so long, and I have had to man up, or rather, woman up, and figure out how to reach my dream.

When I got over my fears and self-doubts, at least enough to get a grip over myself, I realized that I knew much more than I thought I did. I had enough of an idea on how to market myself. I started with my local network and approached people who had done well for themselves in the wedding industry I was hoping to work in. I started collaborations with wedding photographers, videographers, wedding planners, etc. The thing is, just about everyone in this industry is connected with people who matter. One way or the other they all know each other's talents and work.

I definitely needed to make good with all of them to ensure that I was getting somewhere with my prospective business. Over time, my confidence had grown, and I felt more comfortable in my skin. I knew that once people saw my work, they would know of me, and consequently, they would want to work with me. I got through to some magazines, and it was good exposure. But, I wanted to be a sought-after makeup artist, and I knew that I could never achieve it by just growing a local market. If I would get there, I needed to stop playing small, and get myself hard on the track. The fire under my ass grew.

Here, I would like to give my sincerest regards to the founders of social media and google. Mr. Gates, kudos. Thanks to these beautiful people I went full-on research mode, and in doing this, I also fell upon many reviews and success stories. Those fantastic people inspired me, and their stories motivated me. If they could do it, then so could I. I want to tell all of you; never be afraid to bet on yourself. I want you to adopt this mindset, if they can do it, so can you and you can do it just as well. You are unique, and you need to know this, because if you don't even believe this, how will you ever be able to get where you want to be?

One thing about me is that I am a check mark kinda girl. When I need to do a task, I need them done yesterday. To be honest, it is a blessing and a curse at the same time. Where it helps me get things done quicker than anyone else, it also makes me forget to pace myself. It would be all right now when I am young, and I can afford to climb a mountain before breakfast, however, in the long run, it could be harmful. Although, I'll face that when it comes to you guys reading this book; DO NOT PROCRASTINATE! Get shit done, get up off your ass and do something.

Another thing about getting things done fast... yea... they, umm... don't always get done right. Take my word for it, because I have been at the worse end of that experiment. You impatiently complete the task to get to your destination, and you can end up wasting more money fixing your mistakes, and you end up wasting your own time. The thing is, the time you have now is more important than anything you have, money included. You can always make more money, but once spent, time never comes back. That is the most important asset you have.

Anyway, I was talking about the collaboration I did with other artists. I networked with them and I slowly built a network throughout the world, privately messaging them and asking them questions about how they got to where they were. Don't underestimate the power that social media has. In doing this, the first thing I recognized was if I want to be a great makeup artist, my portfolio needs to be, for lack of a better word, fire. Nothing less was acceptable, nor was it even an option.

Through my research and networking with the best in the world, I learned that I needed to make an attractive portfolio. So, I invested in myself; an action I needed to take to become who I want to become. I found a company which helped beauty artists build their portfolio. This was where my savings came in handy, I had planned it precisely this way. I spent it in building my portfolio. It takes money to make money, and I believe that investing in yourself is the best investment. Always bet on yourself. You are stronger and more resourceful than you think you are. Doing a few portfolio shoots, I burned up what little savings I had really fast and panic settled in. This was not because I was regretting going on these journeys, but because I needed to tend to my daily expenditure. I was getting panicky when I saw that my savings were running out. However, this was my starting point, and I knew that to achieve anything I would have to go out of my comfort zone because that is where real growth lies.

It was basically a major gamble I was really hoping would pay off soon. It was something I had to do to get my foot in the door, and in hindsight, I am glad I made all those journeys. The result of making those journeys I had gotten to meet influential people and could network with them and get leads on future job opportunities. The investment I had made on myself paid off!

CHAPTER 5
BE FEARESS AND SAVVY

This is the point of my life where I start the business. Now I have mentioned numerous times before that the hardest part of being a creative person with the attention span of a goldfish is when you have to manage the financial and technical side of the business. That's the part of the business which gets you so bored that you just wanna die rather than actually deal with it. But alas, you kinda gotta.

So, you know how you feel when you have a huge test the next day and you haven't even started studying? That crisis moment is the time when you realize that you can't cover the syllabus in the small time you have... yea it was like that but much more real.

So, in full crisis mode at this point, when I realize I had no knowledge of anything. I'm not the boss, I had never been in that position. The only thing I knew was how to be a makeup artist. I'm a creative person and I can make everyone, feel good and confident. The thing I am not good at is trying to understand the reason behind why the fuck I am supposed to make an excel sheet of everything, or how a website should look like, or anything related to finance and marketing.

I had prepared myself for this, well almost. I had prepared myself mentally and physically to stand all day to be of service to my customers, talk to them pleasantly, understand what they want and try my best to give them the best result possible. Of course, nothing happens for you so quickly. I was naïve enough to think that clients would break down my front door begging me to be their makeup artist as soon as I would start my business. Through that experience, I know that although it is good to aim high, perhaps it is not the best thing to overestimate yourself and end up making an unrealistic timeline.

Suffice to say, it wasn't the best thing to have my hopes so high at the onset of my business. Although, the inner me felt like this was the right time that everything would just smoothly go my way. I feel like I was justified where I was coming from, I had treated this profession as a hobby for a decade, and was now making it into a business, so I never really learned how to run a company. All those years, I didn't need to learn how to run a company, it was just something that I liked doing over the weekends. Going from a hobby to a full-fledged business, I needed to learn all of it, and I needed to do it as soon as possible so that I could generate income and get clients.

Since I have the attention span of a two-year-old, and I was trying to build my portfolio as a makeup artist, around the six-month mark, I was broke. Even though I started out with the grandest of hopes and the best of intentions, my business managed to squash through all those good vibes. The thing is, when you don't have money, even your lifelong ambition can pry on your deepest insecurities. Your brain keeps reminding you, "You aren't good enough." "Everyone was right about you," is yet another insult that I would give to myself. I kept thinking, "You can never do this."

Around the six-month mark, I wanted to throw in the towel and just be done with it. It wasn't as if I wasn't prepared to give it my all. It was just that I was scared that I would fail even after giving it my all. I went through this feeling every hour, of every day and just be done with it. I could get my old job back at the hospital, and be satisfied. But that just wasn't me. I had to give it my all, however, even that didn't stop me from wanting to quit every day. The problem was that I had become sort of set in my ways. I wasn't open to change;

I thought that my mad skills and my personality would be enough to drive the business towards success.

That is impossible, until and unless you know your business like the back of your hand, you never know what to do to bring it closer to where you want it to be. My mind could not accept the fact that despite me being a great makeup artist, my skills weren't enough to propel my business towards success. I would always go above and beyond for the needs of my clients and I have a good personality. In my mind, that was all I needed to be successful, and when I found out that no, it was not in fact enough to be successful, so I used to say, "Woah… what a rude awakening."

A couple of months in the business, I found out that skill was not the only prerequisite for a successful business, perhaps the most important one. I realized that it did not matter how amazing I was as a makeup artist when no one knows who I am, even the people who do know me don't know where to find me, nor was I visible on social media; which was fairly important since social media is an important tool. However, apart from this, there were also other ways to generate leads online.

Businesses have moved from traditional advertising to online advertising. You need to be seen, to be active and online on your profile and you need to be consistent in putting out valuable content. There are new ways and so much to learn on how to advertise in the online world. Being the stubborn mule, I am, I put off learning. Mainly because I have like zero patience when it comes to different things that require time and patience. If something needs to be done, I want it done as soon as possible and tick it off from my checklist. And since I did not know how to go about dealing with the technical side of the business, putting it off seemed like the best possible option. Just to give you an idea of what I needed to figure out, here is what I needed to do now as a starting point for my business:

- I need to build a killer portfolio.
- I need to learn how to advertise and become an influencer;
- How to network and collaborate with the right people in the industry.
- I needed to learn to market my brand and services.
- Be visible on social media; showing my work was not enough.
- Crunch my numbers; I don't even know what that means, to be honest.
- Structure my prices, deliver premium value and create offers that my clients need.

- Figure out the technical side of my business; umm… okay?

One. Woman. That's it. That is all I am. Not a super one at that Just a normal human being. How in the fuck am I supposed to do all of that? Since necessity is the mother of invention or learning, I needed to figure out a way to do all of this. But even after making up my mind, I still could not figure out which to prioritize or where to start. So, I decided to proceed methodically.

The first order of business should always be money; there needs to be enough money to cover the running costs and since my bank account was kind of in a slump I needed to crunch some numbers. I need to figure out what my living expenses were, my business expenses, and how much do I need monthly to survive. When you do this, you sort of get a sad reality check. There is a lot to do and not nearly enough resources to possibly do all of that. So, you need to act fast and get resourceful. After I had figured all of that, I needed to figure out how many clients I need to make ends meet, monthly, before I go completely broke, homeless or worse; back to where I started, my passion going back as a weekend gig. The thing is, when you figure out all of this, you realize that more questions need to be answered. Is my business profitable? I came up with that answer pretty quickly, I had no idea what the running cost of my business was. How many faces and weddings I need to do every month to make the cost, which I didn't know, to make my business profitable. Also, I had no idea what the yearly costs were of my business, or how much the supplies were costing me. Am I even breaking even or I am negative? Turning over a profit was out of the question so I didn't even bother considering that.

Here is where I needed to draw a line. I would not go into debt and lose everything just so I could follow my dreams. That did not seem like a good investment. If that point was ever to come, I didn't know what I would do, so I decided to just draw the line and think about it if I ever got to that point. Even thinking about all of these things was so fucking scary. I was completely out of my comfort zone and everything was insanely overwhelming.

You see, being a makeup artist was something that came naturally to me, and when these things did not come naturally to me, it frustrated the hell out of me. Talking about and dealing with money became very stressful, because it would just remind me how much I had left to do, and just how far behind I was. When you are running out of money and have barely enough left over to cover your own expenses, you get scared.

Then the moment comes when you even maxed out your credit cards to support yourself, and not even the luxuries, just the bare necessities are unaffordable for you, this can make your situations stressful and leave you anxious. I used up all of my savings and used up all the credit I had to pay for both necessities and the business expenses, and that was starting to give me pain in my stomach.

On top of that, it was really mentally harassing. I had a consistent job, and during that time the biggest worry I had was calculating a putting a percent of that into my savings account. That is the biggest pros of having a steady 9-5 job. You don't need to worry. Learning to do something by yourself means that you need to make mistakes and just hope that you aren't making enough that make you go completely broke. The trials and error part of being self-employed comes with such a huge financial headache when you are just starting out. That can cost you a lot, and all you're left with is the hope that you don't make a mistake which is too expensive and that is exactly what happened. Months had gone by, and I still had learned nothing that I needed to enhance my skills as a business owner. As a result of that, my accounts were now in negative balance.

When I say that I still hadn't learned anything, I mean that I was trying, or not wanting to understand it, I procrastinated because I was stressed out with money around this time. I was losing my motivation again and feeling so very defeated. I was worried sick every day. I lay awake at night trying to decide if I should give up or continue. I didn't want to owe anyone or lose my car or my house because of this. I'm starting to lose faith in my dreams and didn't feel at that time worth it to chase my dreams because of the financial burden all I see is fear of failing and in some ways, I felt I've failed financially.

Why? The? Fuck? Was? This? So? Hard?

I had thought that by this point in my business I would have made thousands of dollars, instead I felt cornered and absolutely defeated I felt like I need to make a decision to continue chasing this dream or run for the hills. What happened to that story where the brave girl follows her dreams and she went on to be a success and became a millionaire? Where was the pot of gold at the end of the rainbow?

Instead of being the brave girl who chased her dreams and became a millionaire, I would be remembered as the stupid girl who went after what she believed in and went on to become a failure and lost everything. I swear, it felt like it was game over. I could hear the pathetic tunes of failure ring in my ears and that was that. I tried and I failed. There was no going anywhere from here, I was depressed, had just squandered all of my savings to no gain, and lost everything. I was so depressed that I could not even bring myself to get out of bed in the morning. I hated feeling that way, and I hated myself for putting myself in that situation. I wondered if I should have listened to everyone who told me that this was a fool's quest and that I should not chase my passion, my dreams, creating my reality.

Worst of all, that line I had drawn, where I thought that if I ever went into debt, I would stop and give up, I had even crossed that line. To add to my misery, I was lying in my bed, just thinking of a way to get it together. My passion had led me here, to be a big fat failure. I. Feel. Like. SHIT! Let's face it, it's kind of embarrassing to be so ballsy, quit my job and invest all of my savings, I could never make it. My dreams are just that; a dream. To be honest, I don't think embarrassing covers it; more like humiliating, devastating, mortifying, crushing... yeah, those words would be better suited to describe how I felt. I was actually living out my worst nightmare, and I was paying to live it, of my own free will and accord. I felt defeated as if my life is over and I have nothing to show for it.

You know there are like two levels of broke; broque and broke. Now broque is kinda nice to say. It feels a bit better, but no, I was broke. It was pathetic and very demeaning. When you're in a negative head space, down below rock fucking bottom, your feelings start to manifest in your mind. They are all you can think about. Nothing was going right for me, I was unhappy, confused, and I cried a lot. I think my mind kind of shut down during those weeks. Now that I think about it, it was sort of like a defense mechanism so that I could protect me against those feelings of loss and self-criticism from coming up again.

I remember everything that had happened as if it happened yesterday, but when it came to this, I couldn't even remember how many weeks I was sulking in self-pity for. I remember that all of these negative feelings also affected my relationship. My bad feelings translated to my low energy vibration and that negative energy showed up in my bank account. Thank god for Tyler's words: everything will be okay; not to worry too much; money will come; this is just part of having a business; you win some you lose some; you just started; it takes years to build a successful business; stop beating yourself up; and gosh so many other things I can't even remember.

Now, it may seem like hearing these things are useless, because let's face it, they have no practical effect. However, they have an emotional effect and that is what slowly got me up. I wasn't exactly listening, but his words must have registered on some level in my brain. I was way too proud to ask for his help or even take it when he offered it to me. No that was one line that I could never bring myself to cross. I don't know what changed... but one day; I woke up a different person. I know it seems like the things shown in movies and storybooks, but that is exactly what happened. F.E.A.R. completely took over me. I do not want to be a failure; I do not want to be broke. The point is I want to wake up doing what I love and having the financial freedom. I can have both and not have to compromise between doing what I love but not making money or making money not loving what I do. This was the same F.E.A.R. that took over me when I had left my job, just did not want to settle on something that did not make me happy when I know I can step into my power and do great things. This F.E.A.R. led me to jump ship and leave my job. This was my epiphany and I realized that I needed to jump again.

The F.E.A.R. made me realize what I needed to do again. Same shit different pile. I'm striking out in this business but fuck me if I don't keep playing the game. And this time, I jump higher. I got up, got my shit together and learned all the shit I did not want anything to do with. Back when I wasn't understanding but still trying to learn, those things must have registered on some level, because it came easily to me now.

Soon enough, I was working day in and day out. All those questions I had before I found their answers. I learned how this process leads to premium paying clients that didn't question my price and value and during all that, without even realizing, I went through a lot of self-development. I learned to build a solid business plan, brand myself and in addition to that, I increase my income. I realized that I needed to clone myself so I could save the sinking ship that was my business. Let me tell, you there is no next level of bad-assery than this. However, there were still bad days, but there were a whole lot of good days than there were bad. One minute I would be super high on winning and then the next minute I would be pulled back down and feel like a failure, same as what I felt before. The only difference was a different mindset, I had F.E.A.R.

However, this made me question things, maybe I wasn't right in my head. I wondered if I was bipolar. How was it that I was feeling something one minute and something different the next? What the fuck was even going on with me. Then I realized that I am a female entrepreneur and that is basically the same shit.

The learning curve went on for two months and there was a shitload of sensory overload but in a good way, because I knew that I could take on it. I am also now able to switch my mindset and I'm more determined than ever because I have my business at stake. I've wasted enough time feeling sorry for myself and I won't continue to wallow in sadness any longer. I was being challenged, and that was amazing. Now it's time to implement everything that I had learned and get practical use out of it and let me tell you, it is one thing just knowing what you need to do and a completely another thing to take action towards your goals.

CHAPTER 6
IT'S MORE THAN JUST A PRETTY FACE

Things are finally on track. My marketing plan is perfect, it's reliable, and it's bulletproof. Fuck yea, now it's time to be Little Miss Savvy and slay once again. I have laid the groundwork, worked hard for it, now it's my time to shine!

Yea, not quite.

The thing is, when you have done that first thing on your to-do list, you are just getting started. The success is still several steps away. Now, I had to implement my marketing and strategy to make myself more visible and prominent in the business. I learned it's not about one step and move on to the next, it's about doing multiple things in your business simultaneously. That realization was a big difference in my business. I had gained momentum in the industry and travelled the world for work as an international makeup artist. Honestly, I couldn't be happier and lived every day for my work.

The satisfaction level was just amazing, and every moment spent in improving my business was a moment well spent. After all the hard work I put into making myself prominent, I worked with brides who had extravagant budgets, I also worked with influential people of the media industry, and that gave me the right boost of confidence. Through all my travels I made connections that helped me get more clients and led to even more travelling. Every destination was like an adventure, and every bride made perfect meant other prospective clients. It was like everything was falling into place. I understood how to market myself and grow and scale my business. For that to happen, you first need to find the right niche for yourself. You need to find something you are good at, perfect it over time, and then do that for a living. I marketed myself as a wedding makeup artist and a skincare specialist who led me to a clientele that fit the category I was the best at.

To do that, I had to put in a fair amount of work. When I say fair; I mean quite a lot of work. I researched, read books after books, bought programs after programs to learn to structure my business, and I learned about different methods to attract clients. And these weren't just ordinary clients, these were my dream clients who paid me my worth and did not question my value after just for shits and giggles. They understood that my prices were fair and what I was providing was a luxury service, and they treated it as such. During this time, I continued to invest in myself in different ways, and there was no way in fuck I would give up on this.

The fact of the matter is that when you invest in yourself, or your business, it is a huge commitment. Because you are committing to yourself and even if you break, it isn't something you can just get over. The person you broke that commitment with is your own self, and there is no getting away from that. When you are facing a financial struggle, finding the will to keep moving on is a huge task. It is difficult in every way, and that is because it is there to teach you the value of making something of yourself. If you get everything on a silver platter, then the chances of you fucking it up and not knowing how to get your act together are low. I didn't understand just what kind of incredible things I was doing here. I was taking every opportunity that came my way. I was going all in or nothing, all in the efforts to make my dream come true. I think back to those times now, and I hadn't asked of myself any of the questions I should have, like: Am I crazy? Why do I keep investing in myself when I cannot afford it? Shouldn't I be saving my money for rainy days? I was doing everything in a strategic manner and was growing my network and saying yes to different opportunities and people that I wanted to do business with. People that are ethical, have success proof and can learn and grow from. I had to keep pushing forward because, deep down, I knew that my investments would pay off soon and the reward for my hard work would be huge.

Now came the time I had to put everything I had learned into action. It was execution time, and I was ready to get back to work. I would implement precisely what I had found out from my research, learning from the actions of other successful people online. I had approached quite a few of these people and asked them for advice. I googled and read everything I could get my hands on. I must have gone over hundreds of documents that had anything to do with marketing or making my business a success.

When I first started my research, my initial reaction was, 'okay, this is fun, this is easy. Why does everyone have their panties in a bunch about online marketing?' From what I learned, I was getting traction, visibility, and I was building up my clientele. I felt proud and accomplished that things were turning around.

Since I was getting inquiries about my work from potential clients, which just meant that the marketing plan was working. So, I was ready to launch and put myself out there. Gradually I made progress and income slowly rose.

With the sales on the up and up, I made enough money to earn a considerable amount of my investment back, but it was not fast enough nor was it consistent. I had assumed that I would make a scalable income at the end of the month. Because of that inconsistency, I was always feeling hopeless.

Businesses can't deal with inconsistency, they need to be stable. At least, that is what I thought. I thought successful business made tons of money every day and had clients walking in every minute. So where was the consistency for my business? One day I would have several clients lined up, the next day nothing! I was making money one day, and then the next day I wasn't. Suddenly, I was feeling hopeless again. The inconsistent sales process was driving me crazy. I thought I had fixed this shit already!

Most people who know me understood that I had come close to throwing in the towel. Through all those emotions of hopelessness, I had come this far, and I didn't want to waste all that time, money and energy and drain myself completely. But what about my dream? I couldn't just abandon it. Could I?

Now, most people who are running a business won't freely admit that they are broke because let's be honest, it is embarrassing. But they could still see the stress and worry on my face, and they used to ask me why I was doing this?

Why was I hurting myself and making everything so hard on myself? They couldn't understand what I was doing, why I was doing it because they only saw my emotional and financial struggles. And I realized their line of reasoning, but I also knew that their concern was born because they couldn't relate. They had done nothing remotely similar to what I was doing, and anyone who had done that would tell me to try even harder. I knew that I was on the right track and that was all that mattered. Those people understood the value of passion, which was the entire reason I had left my 9-5 job because I wanted more in life.

The naysayers couldn't see the end of the tunnel as I could. I saw the potential to be financially free and have time along with freedom. The end of the tunnel held the lifestyle I desired. I had a lot riding on this passion. I was gambling on myself, and I had one thought to sustain me through those times. Regardless of where I was financially and emotionally, I had come this far. The journey hadn't been comfortable, but I had the destination in sight. I was confident I would be a success story and for that one thought; I would go on, no matter what. I was implementing and executing everything I had learned, and even though I was making sales business was still inconsistent. I wanted consistent sales and clients coming in regularly. I kept trying to figure out what I was doing wrong or if I was missing anything.

I had gone through this before and thought I can't have this bullshit again. I felt hopeless and desperate, and I knew that I was missing something, but I just couldn't put my finger on it. I was doing everything by the book, as I saw and as I read, but all to no avail. It seemed like my marketing plan was flawed, and this is the kicker, maybe this just wasn't for me. I can't remember it exactly, but I am sure I cried and sobbed. Not that glamorous-cry where they still look pretty while being broken; nope. It was ugly crying. And don't you dare judge me, I had been through a lot. Ironically, I was judging myself. I remember thinking, 'Well, okay... I'm in debt, but it's not that much. I can totally let go of this now. I've proven my point, everyone is right. I need to cut my losses and save myself while I still can.

Yea that phase lasted a couple of days. Now you may have noticed that I have said at many points in this book I would go on no matter what. And then I think about giving up. What you must understand is that you will have moments of ecstasy in your deepest, darkest hours where you just get a surge of energy to go on. And you will break down again.

But what matters is that your heart kicks you out of the stupor of desolation, and wills you to go in the destination is just in sight. Let's just go all the way!

But I knew that I needed help. So, I decided that I needed someone who knows what they are doing, love it, and making a killer amount while doing it. I needed a business coach. And realizing this meant that I had to reinvest, which meant that I needed the money and I knew that I couldn't cut corners on this one. This will not be cheap! I looked at my financial situation again, and I was stretching myself. At that point I had to ask myself, how much am I willing to invest and what is the worst that could happen?

It was pretty intimidating to think I would have to stretch my finances when I was barely making ends meet as it was. However, the inconsistency in my sales made it a necessity. I needed to figure out what was missing or broken. But there was another way, I had to get resourceful. I sat down with a pen, paper, a calculator, and my laptop and figured out how many clients I needed to pay for my business coach and I eventually pieced together enough to pay for her. We got to work. In hindsight, one of the biggest takeaways from getting a coach was that I got my mindset in check. When I realized this, I realized just how mistaken I was in thinking I had a good mindset. I was wrong, and I recognized it more when I got into the coaching program. Realizing this was humbling, and it did wonders for my business and my mental wellbeing. My business got consistent, and I understood what had to be fixed. I revised my marketing plan; I felt more confident in my business. Now, remember, I had conducted my research and gone through pages upon pages of documents and now here was someone who was doing it even better than I was. So obviously, not everything can be learned. I couldn't believe how much more there was still to understand. With the realization came the willingness to put in more work. I had a direction to go into, and I couldn't wait to get started, obviously. I had put in a lot of investment, which cost me an arm and a leg. Gradually I saw some of that investment back, and everything seemed more exciting. I gained momentum again. The last time this happened was more like baby momentum; this was an actual real-to-life momentum. I revised my network with influential people in the wedding industry and got some leads on future job opportunities.

In just over a year, after I left my 9-5 job. I had the distinct pleasure of working at the New York Bridal Fashion week backstage for Yumi Katsura and Pnina Tornai. Became the lead makeup artist at the Versace Mansion. Some of my work has appeared in a few major magazines.

My Lashnoire lashes could sponsor most of these events, and all my bridal clients wore my lashes for their special day.

Once I got the momentum, I started showcasing my work, showing where my work took me. I had a hell of a time doing it. This was just a dose of what I wanted my life to be like; travelling the world while doing what I love and getting paid big bucks. Next thing I knew, I was travelling every two months. I had clients that flew me to Bali, Belgium, France, Netherlands, Spain, and other exotic places in the world. With all this, things got better financially.

My marketing was excellent, and I could see that it was working for me and I could generate clients online. Not for a second did it feel like I was working. It was my passion; I was just doing what I loved. With all of that also came recognition. My peers took notice of me and watched what I was doing, how I did it and my moment of jubilation was when even they asked me for advice. The surprising part was that I could actually guide them. I saw it in their faces; they were actually taking note of what I was saying. It was a great feeling to be taken seriously, and I felt validated.

I realized that I was inspiring them and I got a lot of messages from other beauty artists. They told me how much I motivated and inspired them, and all of that was because of me being open, authentic, and vulnerable. I had finally gotten to where I had clients were flying me out to them, and I was getting paid my worth. All of this did not come easy or cheap. But everyone just saw where I am now and not how I got there. To them, it looked easy and painless, but they don't know the blood, sweat, and tears that went into getting me here. I am not ashamed to say that I had a few nervous breakdowns. What kept me going, clinging on for dear life, was a combination of motivation (to create wealth and abundance in my life) inspiration (to follow my passion and make my dream into reality) and just sheer fucking desperation (of not being a failure, of not being broke, not being in debt).

I do admit any person who is capable enough can give you the tools to build up your business, however, it is up to the individual, at the end of the day. You could have the best coach ever but if you are not determined and committed enough to change your business for the better, you could never achieve your dream. You need to take massive determined actions towards your goals. If you don't have a proper mindset to succeed then it is just damn near impossible to have a breakthrough, regardless of having the best coach in the world. That being said, a coach a key player in your business and can guide you towards success if you want it bad enough. I believe your hard work is a combination of everything and tenacity.

I want to give the message to makeup artists and beauty artists that, having a coach is important to have to assist in your success. Hiring a coach does not mean that you are bad at running your business, in my case I knew by hiring a coach, I'm committed to my success and know she could help me fix what isn't working without the overwhelmed, frustration, and wasted money and time. Not only it changed my life but it was the fastest way for me to grow my income.

To this day, I continue to get coaching so I can continue to perform at my highest level. You need to understand that you don't stop growing, and up leveling. When people start their business most of them are overwhelmed and might not know where to start or where to focus on first. They can end up in overwhelmed state of running in a hamster wheel or what I call being a "busy fool"; there are lots of fears and resistance from these individuals. That is where a coach becomes a key player. I wanted to do extraordinary things in my life and call me crazy, but I held that belief all my life. I just had to believe that I had a higher purpose in this life and I would achieve it so long I kept trying and giving it my all. I had faith I could create success, and that was enough to keep me going. Maybe I should have a unicorn for a pet after all... okay sorry.

Eventually my business was off to a fantastic start, but what mattered was not the start but the journey that taught me everything I needed to get to that start. For the first time, in quite a fucking while, I felt proud.

CHAPTER 7
STEP INTO YOUR GREATNESS

After putting in hard work, things paid off. My business was now better than ever, I had regular clients, and the financial situation was looking better by the day. You remember that destination vacation I told you about in my previous chapters? I finally made it there. I now have my dream job, and I am an international makeup artist who specializes in luxury wedding destinations, having my clients fly me out to their destinations just to get my services. I am charging my worth, making clients happy, I am doing what I love, but the most important thing of all; I am working smarter, not harder.

There is a massive difference between working yourself to the bone and working yourself to your maximum potential. When you work so much that you do not have time for anything else in life, it leaves you with zero creativity and ingenuity; which leads to demotivation. Working yourself to your full potential means you have a set plan, proceeding methodically and logically, this results in that task getting complete. So, you decide for yourself; which is better?

I sometimes marvel at the fact that through all this I never forgot my 'whys.' The most important why was, 'why I wanted to specialize in the wedding makeup; luxury weddings to be more specific?'

It was because I knew how important it is for brides to feel the best they can be and then capture that moment for their entire life through great pictures. I shared their wish with them; I wanted them to look on their special day. When they walk down that aisle or whatever their traditions are, they want to feel they are looking a better version of themselves but still completely comfortable in their own skin, with every eye in the room on them. Even more special is the fact I have a solid business plan as a makeup artist. I know that this plan works. I now get to choose who I want to work with and coming from a place where I didn't have even a single client. This was a huge accomplishment for me. I got to this point one year and eight months after I left my job. These twenty months filled me with pure agony and pain. I cried, had mental breakdowns, and just plain lost it.

As I said earlier, all the heartbreak and stress I went through was preparing me for this part of my life. I knew nothing about running my business or handling the clients, but all that the journey, experience, the let downs, the lessons taught me everything I needed to know to run this business. I have grown so much, both professionally and personally because when you go through that stress in your business, you see patterns emerge in your personal life. Every broken thing becomes something to be fixed, and every bad thing becomes an opportunity to become better. That is what my business taught me.

I feel fantastic about my business and where I have led it to, and where it has led me to. I knew in my hearts of hearts that once I achieved this, I would be comfortable with it, I would have a sense of peace and tranquility, and I got just that. I believed it so strongly that it became the truth. But wait, hadn't I just learned that there is no growth in your comfort zone? I had spent the better part of two years right out of my comfort zone and look where that had gotten me. I was so much better because of it, and I knew that something was about to shift. I don't know how I knew this; I didn't understand why it had to change, but I knew that it was going to. Okay… let's rewind. I hired a coach about a year ago, at that point, and the first conversation we had was where I told her my ambitions and goals. She listened patiently on what I had to say and said, *"Ling, eventually, you need to coach makeup artists and beauty artists."* And I shit you not, I laughed in her face. I was barely keeping it together myself, it was tough making ends meet. Just how in the fuck was she asking me to coach other beauty artists? I looked at her and thought inwardly, 'stop telling me what to do, woman.'

I didn't want to be a coach; I was there to be a makeup artist, and that was all I wanted. I wanted to have amazing clients that I loved working with. She asked me to think about it, and that I would be fantastic at it. I just looked at her, thinking I am here so help me with what is not working in my business help me with my marketing, and help me with my sales and she's sitting there, telling me I would make a good coach. She was practically telling me to change my career path, and I put that away, thinking I never wanted to be a teacher! I wasn't even prepared to entertain the notion that I could make a good coach someday.

Six months later, I have accomplished a lot at this point, my coach sent me a message saying, *"I'm just thinking about you, and I know you are ready to be a coach."*

Wait… what?

No way. That was like starting a new business, so obviously, I procrastinated on this. To be honest, I was thinking of all the work I had to do. I mean I just went through this business and all the blood, sweat, tears, time and money it cost me. I just wanted a minute to catch my breath, okay, maybe more than a minute. I Just put this idea in the back burner and let it stew for an eternity. So, I continued doing makeup because It was finally consistent and generating great income and travelling the world doing what I love. Fast forward a couple of months after that, another incredible thing happened in my life. I was chosen to co-author a book. The book comprised of twenty incredible female entrepreneurs, including me, who would share their success stories with the world.

That book is called "the secret diary of a female entrepreneur." I didn't really know what I was doing. I had no prior experience writing a book, and I didn't know what I was thinking when I said yes. Maybe I was just curious about the idea. I never aspired to be a writer, nor did I ever want to write anything. It was an honor to be named among these successful ladies. My job in that book was to write one chapter and tell my story, the pains I had been through, my struggles, and all the accomplishments they brought with them.

Writing this book made me realize that I was unintentionally giving advice from my own experiences. It was a short step from there to writing this book. It set the wheels in motion, and this is where the inspiration for this book comes from. I thought of writing my book, telling my story. I had put in a lot of effort into making it one that was worth hearing.

I wanted everyone to know about my journey, just as they saw my success, maybe they should also see a glimpse of what it was like being me. Honestly, even better than that would be if any of you reading this book could gain even the slightest bit of perspective. If I could just inspire one person, then all of this effort would've been worth it. I want to inspire others to go for their dreams and not be afraid to make it their own reality. Not to be held back by their own limiting beliefs, or the doubts that they are not good enough. You need to realize that other people limiting beliefs; don't have to be yours! When you are focused and determined, anything is possible. The only question is; how hard are you willing to work for it?

That book that 19 female entrepreneurs and I worked on, that book became the #1 bestseller. This was very exciting for me as I co-authored a book which is now a #1 bestselling book, which by default makes me a best-selling author. Around this time, when we promoted that book, I was also writing this book.

I had promoted a pre-launched for *"Little Miss Slay,"* created a group and implement a 5 weeks weekly live series leading towards the pre-launch date for this. When the pre-launch date came, people were excited and pre-ordered this book. That day this book became #1 best seller as well and I become a number #1 Best Selling Author. I was ecstatic, to be a multiple #1 Bestselling Author twice in one month. It was absolutely incredible. I've done it. something I have never thought I could do.

When the women who co-authored the book with me promoted "the secret diary of a female entrepreneur," I didn't realize how well received it was. I became an influencer in the online space because of many factors that involved the collaboration book and my marketing efforts. Apart from that, I do believe that it was also all the little things that I did and worked on from the beginning of my journey, the small wins and the big wins that made me an influencer and for people to notice That feeling was just something else. People wanted to interview me on their podcast, bring me in as a guest expert, speak on stage in front of huge audiences. It was really special. I had no idea what was going on, and I was entirely out of my element now. I had a different audience watching me now; I was getting tons of messages from makeup artists, beauty artists, entrepreneurs, and people in general. They were taking such a moment out of their lives to send me messages.

This was so amazing because I was finally able to be in a position where I could actually use my own experiences to help other people. It was a humbling and fantastic experience, talking to so many people and helping them out. I learned from them, as one can never stop learning, just as they learned from me. Even better than that some would even ask me business advice. These messages were very heartwarming to read, and I loved them all; for a random stranger to take a moment out of their time to tell me all of that is pretty freaking incredible. It is extraordinary and very thoughtful. I couldn't help but wonder; is this the shift I was feeling? My coach had told me I would be a great coach, so I suppose in a way, it was inevitable. I resisted this calling if that floats your boat. However, now I believe it is my calling. My passion is makeup and looking back now that itching feeling; that feeling of comfortable, this was it. My passion leads me to my purpose. My purpose is to help makeup artists and beauty artists generate great income through their passion by assisting them to create a successful business just like I've done in mine. Yes, I'm speaking to you, makeup and beauty artists, I'm confident I can help you. I know who you are, what you are feeling, I know your pains and struggles. I know how hard it is to generate a consistent income and get high paying clients for the work that you do. Most artists are afraid to raise their price or charge what they're worth because they're afraid that they'll lose the clients that they already have.

That mentality basically boils down to having any client rather than having the clients who are actually beneficial to you, even if it means underpricing your services. I know how frustrating it is to have your desire take a back seat when all you want to do is to wake up and do what you love. The more I spoke to makeup artists and beauty artists, I came to realize that a few people had successful careers as beauty artist. They could only work on weekend gigs, afraid they will lose clients if they charge more. The artists I want to help are the ones that are in the same position as me a few years ago. The artists that are struggling with their businesses, not having a consistent income and the ones who secretly want so much more in their lives. When I do, I love speaking to them, showing them what I've done, sharing my experiences and knowledge in my business. I help them and change their lives and businesses. The more I'm around beauty artists to give them advice and show them what I know, the more passionate I've become. It is the perfect cycle.

I help others, and in that effort, how I can help them with what they are struggling and help them fix what is not working. I'm feeling excited, I get to work with artists just like me. Being able to provide them with what I know and serve them so they too can have the success I have now. It is time for artists to show who they are, that they can make a good living from their passion.

I've always thought makeup and beauty artists are unique I know this because I've been where they are. My mission is to give them the tools to create a successful business. I want to be the one who can show them to step into their greatness and take over the world. Well, not quite take over the world. But ya know what I mean!

CHAPTER 8
BRING ON YOUR SUPER POWER

It has not been a comfortable journey by any means, but by God, I embraced all of it. To be honest, this voyage has harassed me, annoyed me, frustrated me, and angered me so much that I broke down several times during it but at the same time, deep in my heart I was positive throughout it all; although there were days where I lost my temper and even made the people around me go through it too. That was most probably what kept me going. Do you know why this happens? Whenever you are pursuing something you really, really want, it gives you a swift kick in the ass, and keeps beating down on you. Your goal, whatever it may be, crushes you to the ground and keeps you there till you learn to get back up on your feet.

Let me put it in the timeless words of the greatest, Rocky Balboa:

"It ain't about how hard you hit, it's about how hard you can get hit and keep moving forward. How much you can take and keep moving forward. That's how winning is done!"

Do you think he was just talking to his son in that scene? Because I don't. I think he was talking to every kid, every man, and every woman who saw that movie. He was giving us the cold, hard truth of life. Your struggles are your own. You cannot compare them with your efforts to those of the rest of the world because you can never know what they are going through, nor do they understand what you are going through. However, all these struggles have something in common. They are blessings in the disguise of your worst fears. Do you wonder why they are so unforgiving, relentless? It is because they are there for your betterment. You would never have been able to be your best self without being ready to go through the toughest place and come out standing, beaten and battered, but standing tall despite it all. Learning the finances of the business and the emotions you go through while learning about it are very uncomfortable. But, and I cannot stress this enough, the journey to success has been somewhat very eye-opening. When your mind and body are both ready to quit but that one part of your heart goes, 'not yet.' You need that one small part to be the significant part and that voice should not just come from your heart, but from your mind and body too.

If you can't feel that desperation to keep going on no matter what, then you don't really want it. All this has to do with a simple fact that humans are very resilient by nature. More so than we even know at the beginning of our struggles, because after the mental, emotional stress I was under, I did not understand I would make it through. I was just a small-time girl who was trying. That was all I was doing. People look at the level of success I had achieved, and they think I'm something special. That is literally the furthest thing from the truth.

I am just like any other makeup artist out there who wasn't happy because I wasn't working on passion full time. To gain that happiness, I would do literally everything and anything I could. It was just a matter of trying. When you want to do something, when you feel as if you actually cannot live without it, only then will you take that first step. I once thought that that would be the hardest step. That is like middle school kids thinking that once they go to university, it'll be easier because they'd only have to study things related to their field. Yea, good luck with that. Once you take that first step, every passing day becomes harder. You realize just how much you don't know.

You know, I can't remember the number of times, I wanted to up and quit all of it. But every time I was on the brink of doing it, I would hear some small voice in my heart going off, 'not yet.' And I would lie down find some hidden reservoir of strength in my heart. It was not enough to energize me just enough to make sure I went back to working on my passion. And to be honest, that was all I needed.

After you quit your job, and the going gets tough, you think you expected that. But expecting something and being in that situation are two things that are so different that no one can even imagine it. There just isn't anything that is even remotely available which will prepare you to handle your own business. In all honesty, it is a beautiful experience because it teaches you so much about yourself. Things that you could never have found out by yourself, staying in your comfort zone.

People nowadays are really struggling to find themselves and to do that they go camping, try to be one with nature, or try meditation or yoga. To all those people I say; it is amazing that you are at least trying to take the initiative.

In my point of view, the only way a person can learn about themselves is putting themselves out of their comfort zone. Where your comfort zone ends, growth begins. Because at that moment you find out if you're active or not. Everyone thinks that they could handle business and do everything that their minds dream up. But in reality, only a handful of people can do that.

Why do you think that is? The reason is simple. When you get out of your comfort zone and follow your dreams, the reality is a letdown. You never thought it would be this hard. You didn't know how much you still have to learn about everything. You thought you'd be struggling for a month or two, or even six months, and then you'd have a stable business.

Also, if you expected to learn new things, you thought since it was related to your field, you'd be able to pick up on them quickly. Or even if you didn't pick up on it easily, you'd be able to get it once you sat down and concentrated. If you think so, then let me ask you this. How are you going to focus when everything seems to close in on you? When you don't even have peace of mind from a single aspect of your life.

And the cherry on top. You had it good when you were working 9-5. You want to get to your destination, that perfect picture you have in your mind, quickly. But people don't realize just how difficult that is. Just to get to that point in your life, where your dream comes through you need to take care of a thousand and one things before. You need to be capable enough to juggle your personal life and your professional life. And both are such vast topics because within them are a thousand things you need to attend to. Things that need your attention and things you just cannot avoid. Your family, your house, the chores, family events, funeral, someone gets sick, someone has a baby, someone gets married, your boyfriend, husband, children, your friends, your own health, your doctor's appointment, preparing your own food, cleaning up your house, living up to the expectations of people. These are just a couple of the things off the top of my head, and these are only for your personal life. When we get to your professional life, well, that is just fuck all. First, you need to learn a thousand new things to be capable enough to run your own business. But you know the most exciting thing about all of this.. literally, everyone can do it. You need not be special, you just need to be willing not to give up. I do not say this lightly, but the only way; the only one way you fail is if you give up. That is the only way to fail in this world. Because let's be honest, what is the worst that can happen? You spend all your savings learning lessons? Well, what can be better than that? Even the physical and emotional turmoil you feel while learning those lessons strengthens you. Just imagine being the person who is in the midst of the biggest problem and is calm because honestly, they've seen worse. That is the person you become when you face turmoil.

I will not lie, though. When you are going through that, it is fucking horrendous. You literally feel as if you cannot breathe like everything is collapsing down. Suddenly every single thing is distasteful, and you just want to be left alone, and you want company. But when you have a company you want them to go away. You want a solution to your problems, and it feels like the answer is right there, but it is just so hard to get. You literally cannot do anything at that moment except cry your eyes out. You want to scream and yell, but you feel like you don't even have the energy to do that. On top of that, you know that there are matters that need attending to. You don't also have the luxury of a moment to yourself. But I swear on all that is holy. Once you stop crying and gather yourself back together and get back to work, it is like nothing else. It is an experience. It is impossible to put into words because there are no words to describe what success feels like. And you won't know this at the moment, but that is the greatest success ever. The ability to pick yourself up, dust yourself on, put on the mask of confidence and move the fuck on.

That is what all those hardships are there to teach you. They are the test you have to clear before you're awarded the best gift there is; your happiness, through your passion. When you have tasted that feeling of utter and complete devastation, and then you pick yourself up, that is what you'll remember every time you are in a situation even worse than that.

It's kind of like leveling up in life. You started out at level one, a 9-5 job, then level two, following your passion, then level three, level four, level five, and so on and so forth. Every time you level up, your problems become more significant. But the thing is, you became stronger with each challenge you faced. Every issue made you tougher and better. So those problems become easier to handle.

Business is just about that, finding yourself and making a shitload of money while you're at it. And that is another thing you learn about yourself when you are being torn apart, limb from limb. You learn just how little you need for yourself. Sure, luxury is good, and you're immensely happy when you have it, however, when you are accustomed to a particular lifestyle, then you don't exactly know just what you need and what is there for your convenience. When you're broke as in all of your money is going into your business and the critical stuff with none of it being left over to spend on luxurious items, then you understand that you don't need all that stuff. You are a great person deep inside who is just waiting to be found. Every single person has the willpower to make it big and achieve their dreams. The only thing that remains is that you need to put in the hard work. People say that hard work pays off, you may not see the result of your hard work immediately, you may not even see it in a year but you will see it one day when everything is just as you wanted it to be. When all of your wildest dreams have come true, and all of your wishes are fulfilled. All you need to do is to be patient, be practical, and be logical.

The fact of the matter is that, in making a business viable and lucrative, you need to have a lot of things going on for you. One thing that made it so much easier for me when I was just barely making ends meet is when I hired a business coach. Every single one of us needs a mentor, and believe me, even the people who are now running the best and most successful businesses in the world started in the same spot as you did. They may have had certain advantages, some of them did, at least. However, that doesn't mean that you cannot make it in this industry. Your brain, passion, and your art along with a complete determination, desperation, and constant motivation are enough to push you up to limits that you can't even imagine. However, some people might find this disagreeable, to have a mentor, that is. Because they are unwilling to change. One of the best quotes I have ever read in my life, as it is a fact of life, *"Remember that the only constant in life is change."* That is one of the few things that you can rely on or not rely on.

Anyway, if everything around you is changing, rapidly, that is, then how can you expect to be successful if you refuse to change? You have already tried out one method, maybe you've tried out every way you can think up of. Then why pray tell, do you think someone who knows about their business, know about your business, telling you to try something out might be mistaken? They already have a running and thriving business, and they are making money off of it, so they know how to make a business work. The experiences you are going through now, they already went through, and they came out the other side, hardened and smarter.

They're your peers, your betters, and when you can't figure a way out of the problem you're stuck in, be that in generating leads, having consistent sales, or anything like that. They probably have the answer to help you out. I know this very well because at one point, as you very well know, I was in the same position and I learned from my betters. I used what I learned from them and the system I implied in my own business, the strategies and the steps I've introduced to a small group of artists have yielded powerful and promising results. This is the same method I personally used after trying so many other methods and failures; this was the way that changes my life and my business. A step-by-step blueprint for turning your beauty "side business" into a reliable six-figure income while working only 2-8 hours a week.

Discover the 4 Keys My Students Use to Stay Booked with High Paying Bridal Clients and Build a Wildly Profitable Business...Even If You're Just Starting Out and Don't Know How to Market Yourself

When you've tried just about everything and it doesn't work, just know that there is always a way. Even if you can't figure it out, somebody else can, and they have made themselves a living off of it. If you've been in a bind before and tried everything but it still didn't work, you should know that isn't the end. The ideas that might work are always within reach, you just have to know how to get to them. If you know deep within your heart, you were called to make more money from your passion, and do it in alignment with your purpose.

This program will teach you exactly how to make it happen.

- A beginner-friendly, step-by-step blueprint for getting paid $5,000-10,000 over a weekend for luxurious bridal events even if you're just starting out or don't know how to market yourself

  - How to establish yourself as a respected beauty influencer and profiled in magazines, podcasts, and media outlets even if nobody knows who you are yet

  - How to turn your side business into a REAL, sustainable business without drowning in technology, digital marketing, or confusing "business tactics"

  - How to free yourself from being a "slave" to your business by creating more freedom by working less without sacrificing your income

This is not a Get Rich Quick program, sorry to burst your bubble but there is no such thing. I have put this together based on my life experiences and success. What you choose to do with it is up to you. At the end of the day, how much action you take is on you and you only. The fact of the matter is that the 4 keys I applied in my business ensured that I was able to consistently generate greater and greater income. This method can show you the path if you follow these 4 keys process. If you are good at what you do and you are willing to do whatever it takes, to get results for yourself then, these simple 4 keys strategy will be a game changer. When I discovered and implemented this strategy in my business I was able to have a consistent and predictable flow of clients and earn a sustainable income and have the confidence in having a successful and fulfilling business.

The place you're at now is the exact place that I have been through and come out of. I understand exactly how you feel. I can relate to your struggles, your pains, and to be honest, I remember those pains pretty well because I was there just a couple of years ago.

Most of the makeup artists, hair stylists and beauty artists out there who are trying to follow their passion are creative, imaginative and cannot even think about the delicate intricacies which are so crucial in running a business. There are a thousand and one details that need to be attended to and all of them need your undivided attention.

All these details can be so overwhelming and they can make you feel as if the walls are closing in. Do you know why that is? Because you don't have anyone who can relate to what you're going through. Well, all you need to do is look. You have it in you to succeed. So, bring on your super power!

RESOURCES

MAKEUP AND BEAUTY ARTISTS

Facebook Group:

Make sure to join Ling's Facebook closed community group. This is a very valuable group to join for makeup and beauty artists that are looking to learn and up level their businesses. Ling does weekly live on tips, ideas, how to develop a winning mindset, and everything business related.

She also brings in the best experts in the industry. From social media experts to marketing, sales and branding to help you succeed in your business.

This is a place where all artists around the world can support and collaborate with one another.

https://www.facebook.com/groups/themakeupandbeautyartistslounge/

Let's work together

Are you committed to up-levelling your business?

If you are ready to work and be mentored by Ling and want to know more about her coaching program, you can get a hold of her on any of her social media handles below

LinkedIn: www.linkedin.com/in/lingagaran
Facebook.personal*:* @lingagaran

FB.Page::. @MakeupBeautyArtistsSuccessCoach

IG: @lingagaran

BRIDES AND WEDDINGS

Facebook Group:

For brides to be, join Ling's Facebook closed community group. Planning your big day is a very special time in a bride's life. Ling does live weekly on this group and she discusses everything beauty. From skin, makeup and hair.

To help you plan and get insights when planning the biggest day of your life, she also brings in the best professionals in the wedding industry as guest experts.

https://www.facebook.com/groups/themakeupandbeautyartistslounge/

Let's work together

Ling only take 2 weddings a year. This is so she can can give them the utmost energy and attention to her brides.

Website: https://www.lingbelleza.com

Facebook Page : @bellezabylingagaran

IG: https://www.instagram.com/ling.agaran/

LITTLE MISS SLAY